Take...The First Step

FIT AND FASTER

100 WORKOUTS FOR WALKERS AND RUNNERS

---

100 aerobic workouts and training tips to develop endurance, stamina, and increased speed

Lynn Gray
Take...The First Step
RRCA Running Coach

Fit and Faster

Copyright © 2008 by Lynn Gray

All rights reserved. No part of this book may be reproduced or transmitted in any form or by any means without written permission of the author.

ISBN 978-1-4357-5304-4

Dedicated to all my running friends of *Take...The First Step* and my competitors who have helped me become a total runner.

Table of Contents

Introduction 1

Chapter 1: Increase or Decrease the Miles of a Workout 3
Chapter 2: Finding Your Fitness Level 5
Chapter 3: Set Your Fitness Goal 9
Chapter 4: The Beginning: Move Efficiently 11
Chapter 5: The Training Schedule...19
Chapter 6: From Beginner to Advanced Workouts.........................23
Chapter 7: 100 Fit and Fast Workouts...25
Chapter 8: Stretching and Strengthening Exercises.......................37

Glossary 53
Track and Tempo Pace Charts 59
Notes 60

Introduction

The main purpose of this booklet is to allow walkers and runners alike to practice aerobic workouts which challenge their fitness levels. At the very beginning level, questions such as how long, how much, and how fast come up. Answers to these basic questions become even more critical for the advanced runner, looking to improve their overall performance at various race distances.

It is also helpful to note that all running and walking programs need not be a day to day same pattern of distance and intensity. We can add variety to our fitness workouts by changing speeds, alternating rest periods while on the move, and of course varying distances. You will notice that each track workout and tempo workout offers a changing venue of intensity, duration, and distance.

Following a progression of workouts will allow you to gradually adapt to the stresses that running and vigorous walking creates biomechanically. Your muscles, tendons, ligaments will be challenged from week to week. Taking up workouts in a progression and repeating them sometimes for two to three weeks, will allow your body to adapt, so a higher level can be reached without injury.

This book is intended for those who want to speed walk or run for fitness as well as those who want to prepare for race competition. It provides appropriate workouts for walkers who have never trained before and know only a basic walking pace and form. For the more experienced runner, it provides highly developed workouts with increased challenge.

FIT AND FASTER

How to Get the Most Out of this Book

At the basic level, the way to get most out of this book is to practice working out on a regular basis. Thus develop a weekly schedule which includes the days you know a workout can be practiced. Go for a minimum of three days and a maximum of six days, with a maximum of two workouts per week found in this booklet. During the days in between, go with easier steady walking or running. You will want to consider a type of cross-training on those days between your track and tempo workouts.

Without a doubt, the first stage every walker and runner should develop is a mileage base. A base of miles develops muscular endurance and aerobic capability. From that point you can pick out your track or tempo sessions which match your fitness level and goal. (Chapter 8) For example, leg turnover sessions are designed to help you develop a quicker leg cadence, or up and down motion. Many of us get caught in a rut of easy, long distance miles. A continual physical reminder of quick turnover will help leg efficiency in terms of moving more quickly.

When doing these workouts, it is not necessary to follow the order in which they appear on the list given. In fact, pick and choose from among the workouts included, again depending on your current fitness level and time goal you have in mind for the given distance you have chosen. You can always adjust your distance within your warm-up and warm-down mile or miles, and of course the amount of sets performed.

1
Increase or Decrease the Miles of a Workout

There are many variables that will affect what workouts you do and how many you incorporate into a weekly program. Factors such as age, time, desire, ability all come into play and must be considered as you progress. In terms of desire, some workouts will physically challenge you and will necessitate much determination on your part. Your ability level is also important. Adding intensity, which is what occurs when doing these workouts, should be done after you have had at least two months of consistent walking or running. However, key principles of customizing your workout to your needs are quite simple.

In general, you can increase or decrease the mileage of an individual workout by doing the following:

1. Your warm-up: this particular time takes place before the workout. It is based on easy effort walking or running and can be five minutes, or can be up to a half – hour. Likewise, the warm-down, the time after your workout can be modified in a similar fashion.
2. The amount of repeats: for example, if the workout asks for 8 x 200 yds, you can modify it to 4 x 200 yds, and instead of jogging in between each distance, you can walk in between. Or, in this particular example, you can rest for 3 minutes before doing another repeat.

FIT AND FASTER

Within the range of a complete workout, the following example is a sample workout:

Sample Workout

½ mile warm-up, 4 x 200 yd fast walk or run, with a 200 yd recovery walk or jog between each of the 4 fast efforts, followed by a ½ mile warm-down.

Reduced Workout	**Suggested Workout**	**Increase Workout**
4 x 200 yds	8 x 200 yds	10 x 200 yds
Rest 3 min. between	Walk 200 yds between	Jog 200 yds between

2
Finding Your Fitness Level

Your Fitness Level

Each of you will be better served if you first determine your current fitness level. Before you can go a 5K distance or a 3.1 mile race distance at a certain speed, you have to know what your current ability is. A factor which relates with your current fitness level is to know where your resting heart rate is. You must also know your heart rate at a 50-60% effort, a slow easy walk or jog, a 75-80% effort, a tempo or medium speed effort, and an 85-95% speed effort which generally feels like all out and is done at track sessions. Your heart rate both at rest and during aerobic exercise can tell you quite a bit about what condition you are at currently.

Resting Heart Rate

The importance of an aerobic based measurement system becomes important to the walker and runner because it gives you a baseline of the various levels of exertion you should go for during your daily exercise routine. To simplify this is to state that at a slow rate of training we want the heart rate to reflect 60-70 beats per minute (BPM). As you progress with your fitness goals and quest for speed and distance, you may bump your step rate up a notch and in fact go up to 80-90 BPM. At that point

FIT AND FASTER

you are also experiencing deeper more strenuous breathing. This type of training is usually done in shorter lengths such as on a track or a location that is measurable and accurate in distance. Lastly, you can train anaerobic by having your heart rate go above 90 BPM. In this case, you are going for short distances generally under a quarter of a mile and your breathing is definitely labored. However, with each of these three baselines, a training program can be established which will lead to a more efficient heart rate as your progress in mileage and speed.

How to measure your heart rate

1. Establish your resting heart rate (RHR). To determine your RHR you take your pulse when you wake up in the morning, after not moving for about 5 minutes. You simply lay there for a few minutes and count your pulse rate for one minute. Or if you have a heart monitor, strap it on in the morning and lay down for a few minutes. Most experienced walkers and runners will have one below 60 or 50 BPM, and possibly below 45 BPM.
2. Establish you maximum heart rate (MHR). Go to a track, warm-up one mile, and speed walk or run as hard as you can for 1-2 minutes. Or do the same drill up a hill, if it is hot out, so much the better. You may find your MHR to be 170 or as high as 200. Your MHR is genetically predetermined so forget about raising it higher. Keep an eye on it when you are doing fast training, especially in hot, humid conditions.
3. Do some math. When you engage in aerobic exercise you will hear expressions such as do an easy effort, or a hard effort. Or in mathematical terms, do an easy pace at 50-60% effort, or a medium pace at 65-80 % effort, or a challenging pace at 85-95% ef-

2: FINDING YOUR FITNESS LEVEL

fort. These mathematical percent levels of effort are used to figure the training zone for each of these three categories of efforts. The following are formulas which represent these training zones. Each math computation will give you the BPM you can go up to and remain in "the desired zone"

- easy effort zone = (MHR- RHR) x .50 (easy effort level) + RHR = BPM
- medium effort zone = (MHR-RHR) x .70 (medium effort level) +RHR = BPM
- all out effort zone = (MHR-RHR) x .95 (hard effort level-track) + RHR = BPM

For example, suppose your MHR is 170 and your RHR is 50. Your calculation for your 95% level would look like this: (170-50) x .95) + 50) = 164 BPM

4. The realities of effort level. Knowing your BPM then allows you to monitor your training efforts while exercising by keeping track of your BPM over a set distance and or a set time.

Your Current Exercise Heart Rate

Now that you've done some math, it's time to find out what your actual working heart rate is so that you'll have an idea of how hard you are working when you walk or run. To measure your working heart rate, place your fingertips on your carotid artery immediately after finishing a fast repeat on the track and count the beats for 6 seconds, then multiply that number by 10 to determine the rate for 1 minute. For example, if

FIT AND FASTER

your heart rate is 15 beats for 6 seconds, it would be 150 beats per minute. Only count the heart rate for 6 seconds because you are only resting for short intervals of time and more rest time would show a quick drop in your heart rate.

Changes can now be made with your fitness program knowing how to determine your resting heart rate or easy effort, your medium effort and all out effort.

3
Set Your Fitness Goal

As was mentioned previously, a minimum fitness level can be reached with three days of aerobic training for 20 to 30 minutes. But, what if you want more than just basic fitness? Greater aerobic benefits occur when you increase both frequency and duration of your workouts which result in more actual time on your feet. After a few months of continual and consistent training, you may have found yourself completing your goal distance. The goal distance may be a 5K length. Your record keeping will reflect a consistent time frame for completing this distance. Increased aerobic fitness means adding a third ingredient of training; that of setting your own "personal record" or PR for this 5K distance. A personal record goal or a time goal would now mean intensity during your workout needs to be added. A few ways of adding intensity to your aerobic fitness programs are keeping a steady, slightly faster speed on the open roads, implementing one or two of the track workouts, and hill resistance training.

After you have reached your aerobic mileage goal and have determined the frequency of your workouts, you will want to begin on the intensity. A progression of track and/or tempo workouts will give you this component of intensity. These aerobically challenging workouts found in Chapter 7 are listed in terms of ability level and purpose. Beginners will want to initiate from the top of the workout list, and more advanced may begin towards the middle parts. In any case, each workout should be repeated three or four times, or until physical and aerobic adaptation has been reached.

4
The Beginning: Move Efficiently

A starting point all walkers and runners must understand is the importance of duration, or actual distance traveled. Aerobic training for a longer period of time each week will build your cardiovascular system and will help you "endure" longer distances each week. Distance training will build up your physical endurance and your body's capability to take in oxygen, while maintaining the lowest possible heart rate. Distance training also strengthens your biomechanics which includes your bones, joints, and muscles, while adding mobility to each of those physical components.

Let's look a bit more closely at the long, slow distance walker or runner. This person may initiate an aerobic program with a goal of a steady 20 minutes non-stop speed walk or run. With that in mind, he or she could do an out and back course and time their speed while measuring their heart rate to see if the speed is equal in minutes both ways and the same heart rate is kept throughout the duration. For example, this individual will go out the door and for 10 minutes walk, jog, or run, and then return the same way. The goal is to have an even if not lower amount of aerobic time on the way back, while maintaining a consistent heart rate both ways. When that process is accomplished, the novice walker or runner will then add 10% of their distance, and go at it again.

This weekly or bi-weekly gain in distance will continue until the goal distance or near goal distance is reached.

The concept of a goal distance comes down to spending time on the roads. This "gait" practice time results in leg efficiency, a learned form which encourages your neuromuscular system to develop the easiest way of getting from point A to point B with the least amount of physical exertion. Although not the most exciting part of training, it is the most necessary predecessor before frequency or intensity of workouts is added.

You are ready to increase the frequency of workouts, as you get more conditioned and your actual "gait" coordination improve. Generally speaking, the amount of times an avid cardio walker or runner practices their workouts is for a four to five days each week. The beginner should engage on an every other day basis, while the more experienced and aerobically fit can engage in the 4-6 day workout pattern per week. More advanced runners can practice double workouts, or workouts which are practiced both morning and evening.

Practicing "Interval Training"

Interval training involves a series of controlled distances done at an intense speed which challenges and develops your cardiovascular fitness and endurance. The actual "interval" time period is the time of rest or "easy effort" of walking or running. Interval training has tremendous value for both beginner exercisers who walk, and well conditioned runners who desire to improve their aerobic capability. In both fitness

4: THE BEGINNING: MOVE EFFICIENTLY

categories, it improves ones VO2 max, leg efficiency, and aerobic ability. One basic goal of interval training is to elevate the heart rate to levels higher than those used for easier efforts, which results in slower paced workouts not shooting up your heart rate as quickly. Generally your rest interval should not be long enough for your heart rate to go back to normal level.

When practicing interval training, the participant is advised to warm-up slowly with 5-10 minutes of active walking or running. This warm-up period would be followed with basic stretches to prepare the body for fast motion as shown in Chapter 8. Likewise, after the interval session, a cool-down should be completed which is the same procedure as the warm-up.

There are two types of interval training: that of aerobic or tempo pacing, and anaerobic, a bit faster than your 5K time which leaves you finishing seemingly "without oxygen". Aerobic interval training is best suited for the beginner walker or runner due to their lower **cardio respiratory** fitness. In general, aerobic intervals use exercise times from 2 to 15 minutes at an intensity anywhere between 60 to 80%. Those individuals with poor lung functional capacity should start with two to three-minutes exercise intervals, with rest intervals equal to the same amount of time. Thus, if the beginner exerciser can walk or jog one mile in 13:00 minutes or a half mile in 6:30, their interval workout could be 4 x ¼ mile @: 3:10. As ones aerobic capability increases, the aerobic distances can get longer and more frequent, while rest intervals decrease.

Anaerobic interval training is for those who have a higher cardio respiratory fitness level and for those who desire to increase speed, lactate threshold, and overall aerobic power. Generally anaerobic repeats are done on the track lasting between 30 seconds to 4 minutes, and are done at an intensity of 85% to 100% of ones functional aerobic capacity. Rest intervals would equal the repeat time done. Anaerobic efforts can best be associated with speeds a few seconds faster than your best 5K time. Thus, if your 5K time is 23:18 which equals a 7:30 mile, or 3:44 half mile, your workout would look like this: 4 x ½ mile @3:40.

Two considerations for those who practice interval training are the goal distance and goal time the individual wants to achieve. Longer distances require longer track repeats to develop the lactate threshold, metabolic rate, and aerobic capacity for the event. If one were training for a 5K, interval training of 200, 300, 400 yds, or 220, 330, 440 meters would suffice. On the other end of the spectrum is the marathon distance participant. This longer distance goal would necessitate repeat miles, repeat 1200s, or at very least, repeat 800s just below one's 5K mile time which would assist the long distance runner to develop the necessary lung capacity and leg economy needed. The experienced runner also would want to pursue longer distances off the track at intensity a bit below their desired long distance race pace, also known as tempo running.

In summary, when building an interval weekly workout, the following variables need to be considered. First, consider the intensity of the workout, meaning the speed you can maintain throughout the short distance; be it 60% effort or 95% effort. Next, determine how long you want the repeat to last which is based on the goal distance and desired time you choose to work toward. Remember to monitor the amount of

4: THE BEGINNING: MOVE EFFICIENTLY

time your rest interval will be between each repeat while keeping your heart rate up. Lastly, consider the number of repeats you can do while keeping each repeat at an equal time. Here again, the number of repeats is largely based on the goal distance pursued.

The "fast" workouts listed in Chapter 7 can be done at either a tempo pace or at your 5K race pace. Remember, your tempo pace is generally 20-30 seconds slower than your race pace. Your race pace is slightly under your 5K race per mile speed. For example, if your 5K time is based on a 7 minute pace or a 21:45, then your race pace for a mile would be a few seconds below thus a 6:58 , and your tempo pace would be 20-30 seconds more making the mile now equal to 7:20 to 7:30. You may refer to the mileage & time table in the back of this booklet to get your distance and time equivalent for both your race pace and your tempo pace

You can do one tempo and one interval workout a week if you are an advanced runner. If not, one speed session per week is generally the rule. The main difference between tempo and track work is the intervals and speed effort. Tempo running generally is done off the track and on open roads or dirt paths. When doing a tempo run you push the pace just a bit under your goal race pace for a certain time and/or length and follow those speed bursts with a jog for recovery, then continuing on. Track running differs from tempo running because you are pushing into your anaerobic zone for a specific time and length with an interval of rest before you go to the next repeat.

Walkers can handle the workouts in the same way as runners. Push the pace to a speed walk which would bring you to a 90% effort on the interval workout, and slow walk or rest for a minute or so before doing the next repeat. On the tempo workout, the walker will go an 80% effort and go down to a 50-60% effort which means a slow walk between speed bursts. Like runners, fast walking can improve speed, leg efficiency, and aerobic ability. Determine your goals for the correct paces on each interval or tempo as listed on the **Track and Tempo Pacing Chart** at the end of this booklet.

Tempo Workouts with Resistance:

Resistance workouts can be included in tempo runs, and generally require two types of workouts: training fast on tired legs, and training fast going uphill. Training on tired legs is done usually the day after a long tempo session or a long run. Simply speaking, you learn to run when your legs and muscles are tired and full of lactate acid. Tired leg training is mostly reserved for the longer distance runners who must in fact, run strong in a race when their legs are tired. The half marathon, marathon, and of course the ultra marathoners would be most benefited with this type of training. True of any of those goal distances, the fatigued legs should be put to the test on a soft surface such as trails versus a hard surface. This will give resistance from the uneven surface yet will alleviate the feeling of muscle soreness. Distances covered on your tired legs could range anywhere from 5 miles to 10 or more miles, depend on your goal distance.

Hill training is another effective form of resistance training. Hills can vary from a quarter mile up to a half with a 30-40% grade, such as

4: THE BEGINNING: MOVE EFFICIENTLY

you would find on an overpass or a bridge. If you are lucky and live amongst hills, choose a few hills to practice on. Hill training can also be done in parking garages if necessary. Following your run, do repeats up and down the hill. Begin with two or three and work up to ten. This type of training will give you tremendous strength in your quads, help your leg turnover, and save your hamstrings from additional stress while getting the aerobic benefits of track session.

5
The Training Schedule

It's time to put together a functional program which integrates the various training methods you will implement toward your desired goal time and distance. You must consider your current fitness level, your lifestyle and all of its commitments before putting together a training plan. Your training plan for a distance goal should contain a minimum period of 3 months. The day to day training should launch from the once a week long run or walk. It is with this long effort that the major aerobic benefits are derived and which will most benefit your distance goals.

Running and Walking Organizations

Training long distances can be a lonely sport and your hard work gets seldom validated if you go it alone. Check your city or town for a running organization which supports group runs and which may provide track workouts plus offer a few races which they sponsor. A key ingredient for the novice walker or beginner runner is to find a partner. Once you have a partner, you are more apt to show up on a rainy morning since you are accountable to someone else. Also helpful is to find an organization that stages beginner workouts. It is so easy and tempting to miss workouts due to weather, mood, family, work, and the list never stops. A partner or group will keep you on track.

Your Daily Schedule

After finding your support group or person, it is time to put together a fitness schedule that is realistic with your work and family obligations. Generally speaking a three to six month schedule is the rule for a distance goal and more important for a time goal. Your walking and running technique should be in place first before putting yourself on a formalized schedule with a distance and time goal. Before embarking on a progressive schedule it is reasonable to have the basic aerobic ability and the physical conditioning to carry you to at least three miles.

Both running and speed walking fitness schedules generally consists of four phases: long distance base building, stamina workouts at a steady speed, interval training on the track mixed with consolidation weeks of both tempo and intervals, than a taper of 1-2 weeks before the distance event. Within those phases you may want to pursue a cross-training routine such as swimming or biking to reduce overuse on your leg muscles. However, to get the best at long distance walking and running, you have to practice the law of specificity. Runners improve their running because they practice that skill versus replacing that activity with days of swimming and biking.

Base building is the time when you build endurance and your body stays within a 50-70% effort range. Or if you did a "talk test", this is when conversation is easily handled throughout the entire way. Depending on your goal distance and current fitness level, base building can last up to three to six months. For purposes of our discussion, let's figure

5: THE TRAINING SCHEDULE

that you have a good mileage base. Thus your first month or two will simply be used to build up miles.

Following your base, you will want to develop a more efficient pace versus the daily long, slow effort. Once a week add a tempo run to your schedule. This quicker pace generally initiates the second phase of conditioning. Tempo or stamina runs are characterized by a pace which feels like 70-80% effort. Tempo running pushes your aerobic threshold a bit while forcing your legs to move up and down quicker along with your arms. Your lung capacity will increase after a month or so, as will your ability to run more efficiently, therefore reducing your overall minute per mile time. You will have increased stamina in terms of holding a quicker pace.

As your fitness progresses, you may want to throw in "repeats" or interval training on the track, which is the third phase of conditioning. Among other benefits, doing intervals builds running economy. Intervals accelerate your aerobic ability due to moving into an anaerobic zone at a 95-100% effort. You will realize you are in this zone because it will be difficult to breathe while maintaining the all out pace. This forces your cardio respiratory system to develop while improving leg efficiency since your legs are turning over much quicker than an easy pace. Put into practice a few consolidating weeks of both interval training and a tempo run. These two types of workout will quickly develop a better stride, increased lung capacity, leg power, and overall stamina for your goal distance.

Lastly, your schedule should fit in a taper phase or "down time" so your body can rest before the planned goal race. For a short distance such as a 5K, the taper could be less than a week while a taper for a full marathon could be as much as three weeks. Tapering or cutting down mileage and effort is beneficial for the body, and for the mind. Anytime you want to put your complete effort into a race, you want to be hungry for your time goal.

Your attire for a speed walk or run should include cushioned and stability running shoes, with an average weight of over 11 ounces. The stability will lessen pronation and supination, and the cushion will give your muscular skeleton system less jarring. Along with proper shoes, your dress should include loose, yet comfortable outer wear which encourage sweat evaporation. Most walking and running clothes have "wicking" materials which allow moisture to evaporate "on the run". For women, a jog bra with plenty of support is also recommended.

6
From Beginner to Advanced Workouts

Once you have gained the skills of correct walking or running form, aim for a comfortable gait you can hold onto for over twenty minutes. Develop a four to five day schedule and follow it for two to three months thus allowing your body to accommodate the new stresses put upon it. Following this "breaking in" period, you are ready to begin an aerobic fitness program which includes various paces.

First and foremost, consider what a "basic level" of aerobic fitness is. A steady pace of twenty minutes with a consistent elevated heart rate which reflects 50-70% effort is the first benchmark. Most beginners who have not run before will need to initially proceed with a speed walk then jog a set of short distances which gradually will bring them to a one mile distance. An example of this walk/jog interval, would be two minutes jog, one minute walk, and then repeat this process until a mile is met. Then week by week, increase the time of the jog while lessening the walk breaks until you can jog one entire mile. Repeat this process when adding your next mile, until a twenty minute non-stop jog is accomplished. In terms of walking, use the same process and go for the goal of a twenty minute non-stop speed walk. The interval approach is two minutes speed walk, then one minute easy walk. Then precede the same manner as one who decides to run.

FIT AND FASTER

As you begin your workouts, you will want to become aware of developing efficient breathing while on the move. Breathing through your mouth generally becomes necessary along with breathing through your nose. Be aware of the difficulty you may have as you move quickly with your walk or run. To heavy of breathing can cause you to hyperventilate and create dizziness. The solution is to slow down and get your breathing to a point where you can regulate it fairly comfortably.

Also, while walking or running, stay relaxed. Your shoulders need to be relaxed along with your arms as they move side to side. Again, monitor your breathing throughout. Visualize a flow of movement as your arms and legs gain coordination of movement. If you are relaxed, you should be able to practice the various intensities given later is in this book. Remember, before intensity, you must gain endurance and comfortably complete the goal distance you desire. So if your total distance goal is to run or speed walk a 5K(3.1 mile) event, make sure you can comfortably walk or run that distance before adding the intensity workouts listed in this book.

Do not become overly concerned about having a flawless walking or running form when beginning your mileage build-up. Leg strength and leg economy develop and improve as your distance is attained and even more so, as you practice the progressive workouts given.

7
100 Fit and Fast Workouts

Details: Track distances are in yards, goal times with corresponding paces to aim for are found on **the Track and Tempo Pace Chart**. Track workouts are done on a track…tempo can be done on open roads which have been measured or not. If not, tempo should be done on a perceived effort of 80-85% for the set amount of time given on the chart. Note: all tempo or "push" workouts are to be done at your tempo perceived pace, unless otherwise stated.

Abbreviations and What They Mean:

- w/o = workout – a set length and time of running
- r/p = race pace – your projected finish goal must be determined, then find the pace to match it
- BL = beginner level – runners and avid walkers who have an average weekly mileage 20-25 miles
- IL = intermediate level – runners who have run a minimum of 25 miles per week
- AL = advanced level-runners who have run a minimum of 35 miles per week

100 Workouts

Workout level & emphasis	*Distance	Track Interval workout-r/p 90% effort	Tempo or "push" workout 80 % effort	Your experience:
#1 – BL Leg turnover and leg speed	1-2 miles	8 x 200 Walk 200 during intervals	8 x 200 Jog 200 during intervals	
#2 – BL Leg turnover and leg speed	1-2 miles	12 x 200, Walk 200 during intervals	12 x 200 Jog 200 during intervals	
#3 – BL Leg turnover and leg speed	1-2 miles	6 x 400 Walk 200 during intervals	6 x 400 Jog 400 during intervals	
#4 – BL Leg turnover and leg speed	2 miles	8 x 400 Walk 200 during intervals	8 x 400 Jog 400 during intervals	

7: 100 FIT AND FAST WORKOUTS

Workout level & emphasis	*Distance	Track Interval workout-r/p 90% effort	Tempo or "push" workout 80 % effort	Your experience:
#5 – BL Leg turnover & stamina	2 miles	4 x 400, 2 x 200 jog 200 during intervals	4 x 400, 8x 200, Jog 400 during intervals	
#6 – BL Leg turnover & resistance	1-2 miles	8 x 200 uphill Walk downhill	8 x 200 Jog 200 downhill	
#7 – BL Leg turnover & resistance	1-2 miles	8 x 400 uphill Walk downhill	8 x 400 uphill Jog 400 downhill	
#8 – BL Leg turnover & resistance	1-2 miles	2 x 800 uphill Jog downhill	4 x 800 uphill Jog downhill	
#9 – BL Leg turnover & resistance	1-2 miles	3 x 800 uphill Jog downhill	6 x 800 uphill Jog downhill	

FIT AND FASTER

Workout level & emphasis	*Distance	Track Interval workout-r/p 90% effort	Tempo or "push" workout 80 % effort	Your experience:
#10-BL Run even splits	2-3 miles	10 x 400 Walk 100 during intervals	12 x 400 Jog during intervals	
#11-IL Run negative splits	2-3 miles	10 x 400, 1 second faster each one Walk 100 during intervals	12 x 400, 1 second faster each one Walk 100 during intervals	
#12-IL Equal effort running	2-3 miles	10 x 400, equal effort Jog 400 during each interval	10 x 2 minutes, equal effort, jog 2 min between each tempo	
#13-IL Run negative splits	2-3 miles	10 x 400, 1 second faster each one Jog 400 during each interval	10 x uphill, 1 second faster each time on same hill, 2 min recovery	
#14-BL Long distance stamina	2-3 miles	4 x 800 Walk 4 minutes during intervals	4 x 800, jog 5 minutes between each tempo	

7: 100 FIT AND FAST WORKOUTS

Workout level & emphasis	*Distance	Track Interval workout-r/p 90% effort	Tempo or "push" workout 80 % effort	Your experience:
#15-BL Long distance stamina	2-3 miles	1 x 1 mile, 2 x 800, walk 4 minutes during intervals	1 x 1 mile, jog 5 minutes, 2 x 5 min., jog 5 min. between each tempo	
#16-IL Long distance stamina	2-3 miles	6 x 800, jog 400 during intervals	6 x 5 min., jog 3 min. between each 6 min. tempo	
#17-IL Run negative splits	2-3 miles	6 x 800, 3 seconds faster each one, jog 400 during intervals	6 x 6 min., jog 6 min. between each 6 min. tempo, last one repeat go race pace	
#18-IL Long distance stamina	3 miles	2 x 1200, 2 x 800, walk 200 during intervals	2 x 10 min, 2 x 5 min, jog 5 min between each tempo time	
#19-IL Long distance stamina	3 miles	2 x 1200, 2 x 800, jog 400 during intervals	3 x 10 min, jog 5 min between each tempo time	

29

FIT AND FASTER

Workout level & emphasis	*Distance	Track Interval workout-r/p 90% effort	Tempo or "push" workout 80 % effort	Your experience:
#20-IL Stamina and leg turnover	2-3 miles	1-1200, 4 x 400, 1-1200, jog 200 during intervals	2 x 10 min, 5 x 3 min, jog 3 min between each tempo time	:
#21-IL Leg turnover and leg speed	2-3 miles	15 x 200, jog 200 during intervals	10 x 3 min, jog 3 min between each tempo time	
#22-IL Leg turnover on tired legs	2-3 miles	10 x 200, 5 x 100, jog , 5 x 200, walk 100 during intervals	10 x 3 min, jog 3 min between each, 5 x 2 min at race pace, jog 2 min between each	
#23-IL Stamina-finish strong	2-3 miles	1-1200, 2 x 800, 4 x 400, jog 100 during intervals	4 x 5 min, 4 x 3 min, 4 x 2 min, jog 2 min between each, finish with 4 striders	
#24-IL Resistance running	2-3 miles	6 x 800, jog 200 between, 6 x 100, 1 min. rest for each interval	6 x 5 min, jog 5 min between each, 6 x ¼ mile hill, with 1 min interval rest	

7: 100 FIT AND FAST WORKOUTS

Workout level & emphasis	*Distance	Track Interval workout-r/p 90% effort	Tempo or "push" workout 80 % effort	Your experience:
#25-IL Resistance running	2-3 miles	2 x 1200, jog 200 between, 5 x 200, 1 min. rest for each interval	2 x 1 mile with 2 x 2 min race pace within each mile, finish with 4-100 yd striders	
#26-IL Long distance stamina	3 miles	3 x 1 mile with 4-5 min rest between	3 x 1 mile with 5 min jog in between	
#27-IL Long distance stamina w/resistance	3 miles	3 x 1 mile with 4-5 min rest between, follow with 5-100 yd striders	3 x 1 mile with 5 min job in between, follow with 5-100 yd. striders, or 5 uphill repeats.	
#28-IL Finish strong	3 miles	2 x 800, 4 x 400, 2 x 800 with 200 jog for each interval	2 x 4 min., 8 x 2 min, 2 x 4 min, with 3 min. jog in between	
#29-IL Learn 5K race pace	3 miles	12 x 400, rest 1 min. for each interval, keep repeats the same time	8 x ½ mile at just below desired race pace, rest 3 min during each interval	

31

FIT AND FASTER

Workout level & emphasis	*Distance	Track Interval workout-r/p 90% effort	Tempo or "push" workout 80 % effort	Your experience:
#30-IL Learn 5K race pace	3 miles	3 x 1 mile with 30 sec. rest between each mile	5K time trial at desired goal race pace	
#31-IL Increase leg turnover & leg efficiency	3+ miles	8 x 200 with 30 sec rest interval, 8 x 400 with 1 min. rest interval	15 x 2 min tempo pace with 2 min jog each interval	
#32-IL Increase aerobic threshold	3 miles	8 sets of: 1-400, jog 200, 1-400 with 3 min. rest interval	6 sets of: ¼ mile, jog 2 min., ¼, repeat process 6 times, with 5 min jog between	
#33-IL Yasso workout	3 miles	6 – 800s at your predicted marathon or half marathon pace	8 x 5 min. of tempo, with 5 min jog each interval	
#34-IL Pre-race mid-week warm-up for key race	3 miles	5 striders, 5 – 200s, 5-400s, 5-200s, 5striders-1 min. recovery during intervals	10 x ¼ mile uphill, jog downhill	

7: 100 FIT AND FAST WORKOUTS

Workout level & emphasis	*Distance	Track Interval workout-r/p 90% effort	Tempo or "push" workout 80 % effort	Your experience:
35-IL Time trial to determine your aerobic ability	3.1 miles	5K run on measured course, or track if necessary	6 miles at a pace 5-10 seconds below desired goal race pace. Stop after 3 miles for	
36-A Increase aerobic endurance and leg speed	4 miles	8 x 400, jog 1 mile, 8 x 400	8 x ¾ mile with 3 min. jog in each interval	
37-A Increase leg turnover and leg speed	4 miles	12 x 400, with 200 jog during intervals	4 continuous miles, jog 1 mile, 2 miles at 5K race speed	
38-A Increase leg speed and anaerobic threshold	4 miles	20 x 200 with 100 yd jog during intervals	6 continuous miles, with 6 x 2 min. speed bursts at 5K race pace	
39-A Increase speed endurance	4 miles	16 x 400, with 200 yd. jog during interval	10 x 3 min race pace, with ½ mile tempo between each 3 min.	

33

FIT AND FASTER

Workout level & emphasis	*Distance	Track Interval workout-r/p 90% effort	Tempo or "push" workout 80 % effort	Your experience:
40-A Increase stamina	4-5 miles	12-15 x 400 with a 2 min rest during intervals	10K at tempo pace, followed by 6 x 2 min. race pace, with 30 sec. rest during intervals	
41-A Increase stamina and leg speed	4-5 miles	20 x 200, with 1 min. rest during intervals	8 continuous miles at 5 seconds below desired long distance goal race pace	
42-A Yasso workout	5 miles	10 x 800 at your predicted marathon or half marathon pace	10-12 continuous miles, run 5 seconds below desired goal race pace	
43-A Increase leg speed and endurance	5 miles	20 x 400 with 400 jog during each interval	20 x 5 min. with 5 min jog during each interval	
44-A Finish strong on tired legs	5 miles	15 x 400 with 200 jog during each interval, reduce each lap by 1-2 seconds	6 continuous miles, then 10 ¼ mile hill repeats, jog downhill for recovery	

7: 100 FIT AND FAST WORKOUTS

Workout level & emphasis	*Distance	Track Interval workout-r/p 90% effort	Tempo or "push" workout 80 % effort	Your experience:
45-A Predict goal race time	6 miles	10K at 5K race pace	12 continuous miles, run 5 seconds below desired long distance goal race pace	
46-A Increase leg speed-stamina	6 miles	24 x 200, with 2 min. rest during intervals	10 continuous miles, with 10 x 1 min. race pace spurts along the way	
48-A Increase endurance	6 miles	3 x 2 mile with 400 jog during each interval	6 x 2 mile with 5 min. jog during each interval	
49-A Increase leg speed	5 miles	5 x 1 mile with 2 min. rest during each interval	10 x 1 mile, with 5 min. jog during each interval	
50-A Increase stamina & endurance	6 miles	10 x 200, 8 x 400, 6 x 800	10 continuous miles followed with 8-10 ¼ mile hill repeats, jog downhill for recovery	

8
Stretching and Strengthening Exercises

The stretching exercises shown below are done after warming up with a five minute walk or jog and following your workout.

Back and Quadriceps Stretch

Kneel on both knees, sit on the heels, with your trunk bent forward over the thighs and arch your back as much as possible. Extend your arms forward to their full length with your palms on the floor and place your head down between the arms as far as possible.

Effect: stretches both the quadriceps and back muscle groups

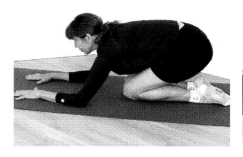
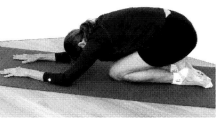

Core Stretch

Lay face down on a mat with your stomach completely on the floor and your legs slightly apart. Place your palms under your shoulders so that the tips of your middle fingers are directly under your shoulder joints. Hold your elbows against your body, drawing your shoulder blades back. While pressing down with your palms, slowly lift your trunk off the floor, keeping your chin down, vs. your head arched back.

Effect: Adds flexibility to the upper back and stretches the front of the body.

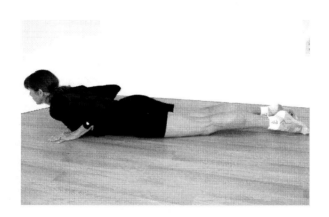

8: STRETCHING AND STRENGTHENING EXERCISES

Shoulder Stretch

Stand tall with your ankles and front toes touching together with your pelvis gently tucked in. Inhale and stretch your arms overhead while interlocking your fingers.

Effect: An awareness of your posture is developed. Hyperextension adds flexibility and your overall sense of balance are improved.

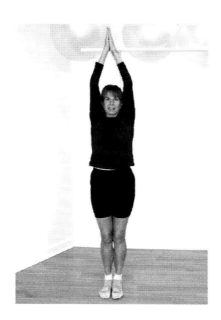

Hamstring Stretch

Sit on the ground, flexing your trunk forward onto the thighs as much as possible, with knees slightly bent or straight if possible. Try to grasp the outer edges of your feet. Place the head down between the arms as far as possible. Hold for 60 seconds

Effect: The hamstrings are stretched as well as the calves and arms.

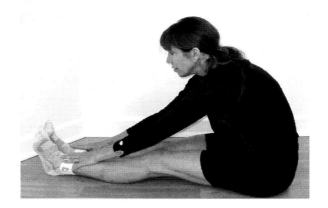

8: STRETCHING AND STRENGTHENING EXERCISES

Groin Stretch

In a sitting position, place the soles of the feet together, bringing the heels as close to the buttocks as possible. With the elbows placed inside the knees, grab the ankles and press your legs down gently with the elbows. Push the knees down toward the floor while flexing the spine forward and pulling the forehead toward the toes for 30 seconds.

Effect: A deep stretch of the inner thighs and hip rotators of the outer thigh.

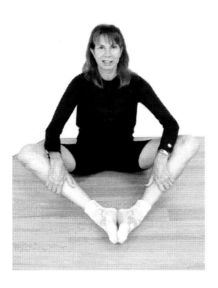

Gastronomies Stretch

Stand approximately 3 to 4 feet from a vertical surface such as a wall or upright support. Incline the straight body forward to an angle of approximately 65 degrees, supporting the body with the extended arms; palms flat against the surface. The calves can be stretched deeper by having the balls of the feet on a 2-inch elevation such as a phone book or two-by-four. Hold for 30-60 seconds

Effect: This stretch is designed to train the calf muscle and Achilles tendon lengthens which will reduce tightness.

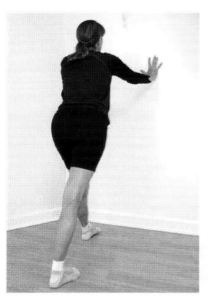 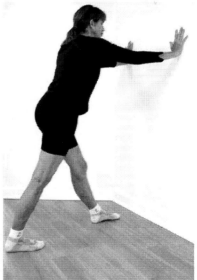

8: STRETCHING AND STRENGTHENING EXERCISES

Forward Bend

Place feet hip length apart and have your heels firmly planted on the ground facing forward. Bend your torso until both of your hands and feet can be planted on the ground with fingers spreading straight out. Lift your pelvis up toward the ceiling. Allow your head and neck to drop down as the forward bending takes place. Hold this position for 30 seconds.

Effect: This yoga pose stretches all the muscles in the backs of the calves and thighs, the shoulders, the belly, and the back. It strengthens the arms and relieves neck tension.

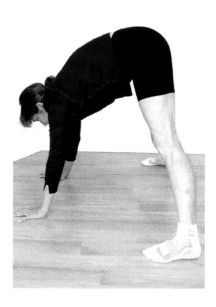

Strengthening Exercises

Step – Ups

On a step stool or bench knee high, step up with your right foot up on the stool then down, landing in both cases, flat footed. Do entire motion quickly to simulate the walking and running movement. Work up to 25 repeats on each leg. Increase challenge with 1 or 2 lb ankle weights.

Effect: Repetitive quick up and down leg motion brings about faster leg turnover and adds to overall leg power.

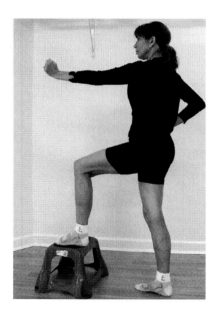

8: STRETCHING AND STRENGTHENING EXERCISES

Abdominal Curls

Lying on your back, knees bent, with feet on the floor and hands crossed in front, curl the upper trunk and hands as close to the knees as possible. Be careful to lead with your chin so as to not bend and stress your neck and back muscles. Repeat 25 times. With the same laying down position, twist the trunk to the left as you go up aiming your left crossed arm to touch your right leg. Repeat 25 times. Reverse twist to the right. Repeat 25 times.

Effect: The abdominals become strong enough to stabilize the pelvis giving your "core" a stronger center resulting in better posture.

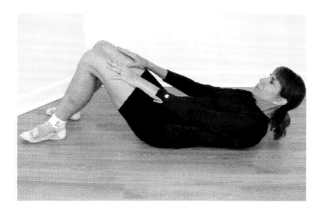

Core Circling

Stand hip length apart, arms free at the sides. Circle the trunk 4 times to the left and then 4 times to the right.

Effect: Movement of the hip flexors increases flexibility and allows a greater range of motion as you walk or run.

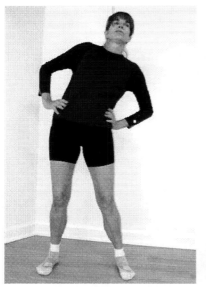 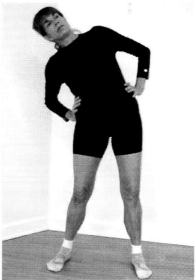

8: STRETCHING AND STRENGTHENING EXERCISES

Arm Swings

Stand hip width apart, moving both arms sideward to the left as far as they can go, while rotating the core in the same direction. Repeat to the right. Keep hands in a loose fist. Keep your feet in place. Repeat 20 to 30 repetitions.

Effect: Movement of the hip flexors and the trunk area will add flexibility to your torso area plus strengthen your shoulders and arms.

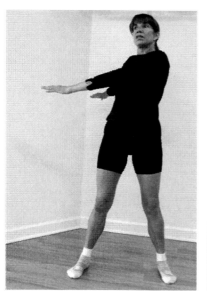 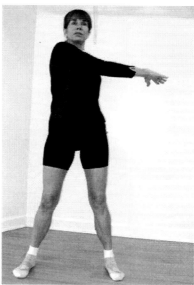

47

Toe Raises

Place your feet less than hip width apart. Rock up on the balls of the feet as high as possible as return back onto the heels. Next roll over onto the outer borders of the feet and then inwards as far as possible onto the inner borders. Repeat the complete sequence from the beginning. Repeat 8-10 repetitions.

Effect: The ankles will become stronger and more flexible. The toe off movement while walking and running will become more natural.

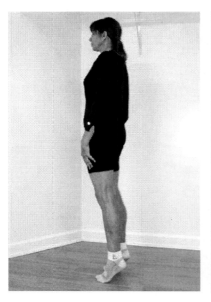 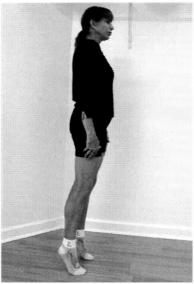

8: STRETCHING AND STRENGTHENING EXERCISES

Arm Side Swings

Place your feet in a small stride stance. Bend your arms and cup your hands around a one lb. weight. Mimic the back and forth flow of swinging your arms as you would while running, keeping your arms swinging close to each respective side part of the body. Vary the weights up to 5 lbs. Repeat both right and left arm swing 25 times,

Effect: Increased efficiency with arm movement while walking or running will result. The quicker the arms move, the quicker the body will be propelled forward.

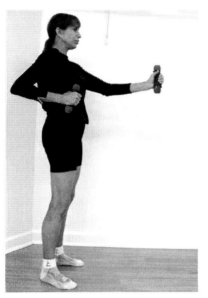 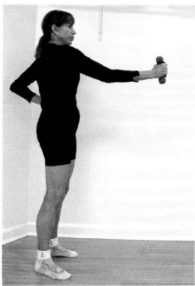

Half Squat

Place your feet in a small stride stance with hands on hips, while keeping the core straight and pelvis slightly tucked in. Then raise the heels slightly off the ground, bending both knees to a half-squat position. Hand weights from 1-5 lbs can be used while doing repetitions. Do not allow your knees to bend beyond the front of your feet. With a moderate tempo pace, repeat 15 to 20 times.

Effect: Strength in your quadriceps and calves will result. Increased flexibility will occur in the Achilles tendon area and calf muscles.

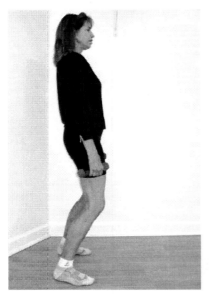
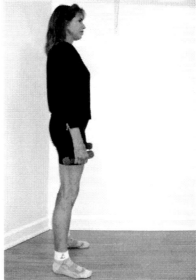

8: STRETCHING AND STRENGTHENING EXERCISES

Pectoral Back Swings

Place your feet hip length apart with arms raised sideward, both bent in at the elbows at shoulder height, palms cupped and facing inward. Slowly and steadily bring both bent arms back as far as possible so as to form a V in your scapular of your back. Repeat 10 times. Challenge will be if 1 to 2 lb weights are added.

Effect: These swings add strength in the shoulders and arm muscle groups and core while increasing balance and posture while standing, walking, or running

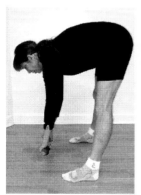 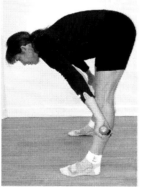 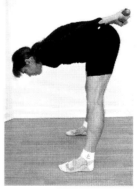

Glossary

Abbreviations and what they mean:

w/o = workout – a set length and time of running

r/p = race pace – your projected finish goal must be determined, then find the pace to match it

BL = beginner level – runners and avid walkers who have an average weekly mileage 20-25 miles

IL = intermediate level – runners who have run a minimum of 25 miles per week

AL = advanced level-runners who have run a minimum of 50 miles per week

Aerobic: exercise which allows adequate oxygen to be delivered into the cells to meet the energy output required

Anaerobic: an effort where breathing is next to impossible due to the fast exertion and your lung capacity being at its maximum

ATP: is also known as adenosine triphosphate and is the body's energy source. The quicker the cell produces ATP the more the cell can function before it fatigues. Aerobic and anaerobic training both help muscle cells replenish the amount of ARP stored.

Cardio respiratory fitness: The capacity of the lungs to exchange oxygen and carbon dioxide with the blood and the circulatory system's ability to transport blood and nutrients to metabolically active tissues for sustained periods without total fatigue.

Cardio respiratory endurance: having the ability to sustain aerobic activity for a prolonged period of time

Core: refers to the "trunk area" which includes the stomach and chest The strong core becomes critical in all sports since it provides balance and ads coordination to both arms and legs

Duration: the amount of time you are engaged in your aerobic workout

Effort based running: This is a perceived personal effort you put forth when you do not have a set measured distance and/or a set time. It is common to walk or run a "medium effort" meaning 70-80% of your heart rate, or a "hard effort" meaning 85%-90% of your heart rate.

Endurance: The amount of time and/or distance you can sustain at a given aerobic effort without total muscle fatigue.

Frequency: the amount of times per week and/or per day you are engaged in your aerobic workout

Interval: a given amount of time and/or distance for recovery between distances given for race pace or tempo pace

Heart rate: The number of times the heart beats per minute(bpm)

GLOSSARY

Intensity: the addition of resistance while engaged in your aerobic activity; a most common example is adding interval workouts to your program

Jog: a slow movement of running which accommodates recovery; usually done at 50-55% of your heart rate   Jogging is also a term referred to for beginners; meaning, learning to go slow while building distance.

Law of specificity: an individual can become both functional and efficient of any given movement, as long as that movement is trained and practiced over and over again.

Lactic acid: is a by product of anaerobic ATP production which when increased in your muscles, results in a reduction of contraction or functioning of the muscle

Leg turnover: refers to the ability for you to run quickly by increasing your ability to run fast due to your legs moving up and down with the most speed your coordination will allow

Negative splits: at a given distance, when repeated, that distance will be run or walked a few seconds fast them the previous given distance

Personal Record: is also known by the acronym of PR. A personal record is a lower time barrier you make on a given goal distance

Pronation: is caused by a weak arch, making much of your weight fall toward the inside of the foot

55

Race Pace: is an aerobic and anaerobic effort which equals to 90 – 95% of your heart rate

Resistance: adding additional stress to legs while running; examples are: uphill running, striders or 100 yd. dashes on tired legs, or running after biking a given distance

Resting heart rate: is measured most accurately just before arising out of bed, and can be found on the larger carotid artery of the side of the larynx or at the radial pulse on the wrist

Speed walk: an aerobic effort which requires active arms and legs moving at a brisk rate; sometimes referred to as cardio walking

Split: a given distance with a given time at a track

Stamina: the ability to hold a continuous medium to hard effort for a distance which puts you in a heart rate range of 80 – 90%

Striders: running approximately 100 yds with the following process in mind: 1st 25 yds slow for form, next 25 yds medium effort, last 25 yds run all out at 90-95% effort

Supination: is caused by a weak arch, making much of your weight fall toward the outside of the foot. This continual foot strike causes a wear pattern on the outside bottom of your walking or running shoe.

GLOSSARY

Taper: a term referred to when the speed walker or runner cuts down mileage and intensity prior to a planned distance goal event

Tempo: or "stamina run" is a longer distance aerobic effort which equals to 75% - 80% of your heart rate

Workout: this term refers to the actual length, time, and effort for each distance given

Yasso workout: Based on the theory of Bart Yasso that when you run up to 10-800's at a given time, you can predict your marathon time. Thus, 10 x 800 @ 4:02 will equal to a 4:02 marathon time…given your distance training has been done.

Track and Tempo Pace Charts

Est. full marathon time	Est. 1/2 marathon time	10K	5K	race pace mile	tempo mile	1/2 mile RP	1/4 mile RP	½ mile tempo	¼ mile tempo
6:02	2:59	1:24	42:50	13:40	14:40	6:50	3:20	7:20	3:40
5:51	2:55	1:22	41:20	13:20:	14:20:	6:45	3:20	7:15	3:35
5:45	2:51	1:20	40:00	13:00	14:00	6:20	3:10	6:50	3:25
5:15	2:37	1:15	37:40	12:00	13:00	6:00	3:00	6:30	3:15
5:10	2:36	1:12	36:50	11:50	12:50	5:50	2:55	6:20	3:10
4:48	2:24	1:09	34:20	11:00	12:00	5:45	2:50	6:15	3:05
4:31	2:15	1:04	32:10	10:20	11:20	5:10	2:35	6:35	2:50
4:23	2:11	1:01	30:55	10:00	11:00	5:00	2:30	5:30	2:45
4:15	2:07	1:00	30:20	9:45	10:450	4:56	2:28	5:26	2:43
4:09	2:04	59:00	29:30:	9:30	10:30	4:50	2:25	5:20	2:40
4:04	2:02	57:50	28:59	9:20	10:20	4:40	2:20	5:10	2:35
3:56	1:58	55:00	27:57	9:00	10:00	4:30	2:15	5:00	2:30
3:51	1:56	54:32	27:26	8:50	9:50	4:24	2:12	4:34	2:27
3:47	1:53	53:50	26:55	8:40	9:40	4:20	2:10	4:50	2:25

FIT AND FASTER

Est. full marathon time	Est. 1/2 marathon time	10K	5K	race pace mile	tempo mile	1/2 mile RP	1/4 mile RP	1/2 mile tempo	¼ mile tempo
3:42	1:51	52:48	26:24	8:30	9:30	4:14	2:07	4:44	2:22
3:38	1:49	51:46	25:53	8:20	9:20	4:10	2:05	4:35	2:20
3:34	1:46	50:44	25:22	8:10	9:10	4:04	2:02	4:32	2:17
3:29	1:44	49:42	24:51	8:00	9:00	4:00	2:00	4:30	2:15
3:25	1:43	48:40	24:20	7:50	8:50	3:54	1:57	4:24	2:12
3:21	1:39	47:38	23:49	7:40	8:40	3:50	1:55	4:20	2:10
3:16	1:38	46:36	23:18	7:30	8:30	3:44	1:52	4:14	2:07
3:12	1:35	45:34	22:47	7:20	8:20	3:40	1:50	4:10	2:05
3:07	1:33	44:42	22:16	7:10	8:10	3:34	1:47	4:04	2:02
3:03	1:31	43:30	21:45	7:00	8:00	3:30	1:45	4:00	2:00
2:59	1:28	42:28	21:44	6:50	7:50	3:24	1:42	3:54	1:52
2:54	1:27	41:26	20:43	6:40	7:40	3:20	1:40	3:50	1:55
2:50	1:25	40:24	20:12	6:30	7:30	3:14	1:37	3:44	1:52
2:46	1:23	39:22	19:41	6:20	7:20	3:10	1:35	3:40	1:52

Notes

FIT AND FASTER

NOTES

FIT AND FASTER

NOTES

FIT AND FASTER

NOTES

FIT AND FASTER

NOTES

About the Author

Lynn Gray is a recognized RRCA certified running coach who resides and coaches in Tampa, Florida. Lynn has been a runner for over forty years, an age group winner for thirty years and has completed over eighty marathons, including ten Boston Marathons. She is also the recipient of the USA Track and Field Masters 5K winner and numerous Master and Grandmaster awards.

Lynn is the founder and President of a running organization called, Take…The First Step which currently motivates over a hundred or more women and men to become physically active. She has been a running coach for twelve years and has training hundreds of participants of all ages and ability levels. Her training programs include KIDS© running, Walk to Run©, My First 5K, Get SLIM©, and numerous other programs which help both the beginner and experienced exerciser get into top shape.

This author has been a competitor most of her life with over 1,200 parachute jumps involving acrobatics and accuracy, a brown belt in Martial Arts, and is currently working on completing the Fifty States marathon challenge. Lynn believes in helping the participant in establishing a life of permanent fitness through her various agility and aerobic ability programs. She currently trains both men and women from the contents of this book.

Get personal tips from the author to customize your training and enhance your results.
www.TheFirstStepPrograms.com   E-Mail: LGray88@yahoo.com